Table of Contents

50 Foods That Are Super Healthy

It's easy to wonder which foods are healthiest.

A vast number of foods are both healthy and tasty. By filling your plate with fruits, vegetables, quality protein, and other whole foods, you'll have meals that are colorful, versatile, and good for you.

Here are 50 incredibly healthy foods. Most of them are surprisingly delicious.

1–6: Fruits and berries

Fruits and berries are among the world's most popular health foods.

These sweet, nutritious foods are very easy to incorporate into your diet because they require little to no preparation.

1. Apples

Apples are high in fiber, vitamin C, and numerous antioxidants. They are very filling and make the perfect snack if you find yourself hungry between meals.

2. Avocados

Avocados are different than most fruits because they are loaded with healthy fats instead of carbs. Not only are they creamy and tasty but also high in fiber, potassium, and vitamin C.

3. Bananas

Bananas are among the world's best sources of potassium. They're also high in vitamin B6 and fiber, as well as convenient and portable.

4. Blueberries

Blueberries are not only delicious but also among the most powerful sources of antioxidants in the world.

5. Oranges

Oranges are well known for their vitamin C content. What's more, they're high in fiber and antioxidants.

6. Strawberries

Strawberries are highly nutritious and low in both carbs and calories.

They are loaded with vitamin C, fiber, and manganese and are arguably among the most delicious foods in existence.

Other healthy fruits

Other health fruits and berries include cherries, grapes, grapefruit, kiwifruit, lemons, mango, melons, olives, peaches, pears, pineapples, plums, and raspberries.

7. Eggs

Eggs are among the most nutritious foods on the planet.

They were previously demonized for being high in cholesterol, but new studies show that they're perfectly safe and healthy.

8–10: Meats

Unprocessed, gently cooked meat is one of the most nutritious foods you can eat.

8. Lean beef

Lean beef is among the best sources of protein in existence and loaded with highly bioavailable iron. Choosing the fatty cuts is fine if you're on a low-carb diet.

9. Chicken breasts

Chicken breast is low in fat and calories but extremely high in protein. It's a great source of many nutrients. Again, feel free to eat fattier cuts of chicken if you're not eating that many carbs.

10. Lamb

Lambs are usually grass-fed, and their meat tends to be high in omega-3 fatty acids.

11–15: Nuts and seeds

Despite being high in fat and calories, nuts and seeds may help you lose weight.

These foods are crunchy, filling, and loaded with important nutrients that many people don't get enough of, including magnesium and vitamin E.

They also require almost no preparation, so they're easy to add to your routine.

11. Almonds

Almonds are a popular nut loaded with vitamin E, antioxidants, magnesium, and fiber. Studies show that almonds can help you lose weight and improve metabolic health.

12. Chia seeds

Chia seeds are among the most nutrient-dense foods on the planet. A single ounce (28 grams) packs 11 grams of fiber and significant amounts of magnesium, manganese, calcium, and various other nutrients.

13. Coconuts

Coconuts are loaded with fiber and powerful fatty acids called medium-chain triglycerides (MCTs).

14. Macadamia nuts

Macadamia nuts are very tasty. They're much higher in monounsaturated fats and lower in omega-6 fatty acids than most other nuts.

15. Walnuts

Walnuts are highly nutritious and loaded with fiber and various vitamins and minerals.

16–25: Vegetables

Calorie for calorie, vegetables are among the world's most concentrated sources of nutrients.

There's a wide variety available, and it's best to eat many different types every day.

16. Asparagus

Asparagus is a popular vegetable. It's low in both carbs and calories but loaded with vitamin K.

17. Bell peppers

Bell peppers come in several colors, including red, yellow, and green. They're crunchy and sweet, as well as a great source of antioxidants and vitamin C.

18. Broccoli

Broccoli is a cruciferous vegetable that tastes great both raw and cooked. It's an excellent source of fiber and vitamins C and K and contains a decent amount of protein compared with other vegetables.

19. Carrots

Carrots are a popular root vegetable. They are extremely crunchy and loaded with nutrients like fiber and vitamin K.

Carrots are also very high in carotene antioxidants, which have numerous benefits.

20. Cauliflower

Cauliflower is a very versatile cruciferous vegetable. It can be used to make a multitude of healthy dishes — and also tastes good on its own.

21. Cucumber

Cucumbers are one of the world's most popular vegetables. They're very low in both carbs and calories, consisting mostly of water. However, they contain a number of nutrients in small amounts, including vitamin K.

22. Garlic

Garlic is incredibly healthy. It contains bioactive organosulfur compounds that have powerful biological effects, including improved immune function.

23. Kale

Kale has become increasingly popular because it's incredibly high in fiber, vitamins C and K, and a number of other nutrients. It adds a satisfying crunch to salads and other dishes.

24. Onions

Onions have a very strong flavor and are very popular in many recipes. They contain a number of bioactive compounds believed to have health benefits.

25. Tomatoes

Tomatoes are usually categorized as a vegetable, although they are technically a fruit. They are tasty and loaded with nutrients like potassium and vitamin C.

More healthy vegetables

Most vegetables are very healthy. Others worth mentioning include artichokes, Brussels sprouts, cabbage, celery, eggplant, leeks, lettuce, mushrooms, radishes, squash, Swiss chard, turnips, and zucchini.

26–31: Fish and seafood

Fish and other seafood tend to be very healthy and nutritious.

They're especially rich in omega-3 fatty acids and iodine, two nutrients in which most people are deficient.

Studies show that people who eat the highest amounts of seafood — especially fish — tend to live longer and have a lower risk of many illnesses, including heart disease, dementia, and depression.

26. Salmon

Salmon is a type of oily fish that's incredibly popular due to its excellent taste and high amount of nutrients, including protein and omega-3 fatty acids. It also contains some vitamin D.

27. Sardines

Sardines are small, oily fish that are among the most nutritious foods you can eat. They boast sizable amounts of most nutrients that your body needs.

28. Shellfish

Shellfish ranks similarly to organ meats when it comes to nutrient density. Edible shellfish include clams, mollusks, and oysters.

29. Shrimp

Shrimp is a type of crustacean related to crabs and lobsters. It tends to be low in fat and calories but high in protein. It's also loaded with various other nutrients, including selenium and vitamin B12.

30. Trout

Trout is another type of delicious freshwater fish, similar to salmon.

31. Tuna

Tuna is very popular in Western countries and tends to be low in fat and calories while high in protein. It's perfect for people who need to add more protein to their diets but keep calories low.

However, you should make sure to buy low-mercury varieties.

32–34: Grains

Although grains have gotten a bad rap in recent years, some types are very healthy.

Just keep in mind that they're relatively high in carbs, so they're not recommended for a low-carb diet.

32. Brown rice

Rice is one of the most popular cereal grains and is currently a staple food for more than half of the world's population. Brown rice is fairly nutritious, with a decent amount of fiber, vitamin B1, and magnesium.

33. Oats

Oats are incredibly healthy. They are loaded with nutrients and powerful fibers called beta glucans, which provide numerous benefits.

34. Quinoa

Quinoa has become incredibly popular among health-conscious individuals in recent years. It's a tasty grain that's high in nutrients, such as fiber and magnesium. It is also an excellent source of plant-based protein.

35–36: Breads

Many people eat a lot of highly processed white bread.

For those trying to adopt a healthier diet, it can be extremely challenging to find healthy breads. Even so, options are available.

35. Ezekiel bread

Ezekiel bread may be the healthiest bread you can buy. It's made from organic, sprouted whole grains, as well as several legumes.

36. Homemade low-carb breads

Overall, the best choice for bread may be that which you can make yourself. Here's a list of 15 recipes for gluten-free, low-carb breads.

37–40: Legumes

Legumes are another food group that has been unfairly demonized.

While it's true that legumes contain antinutrients, which can interfere with digestion and absorption of nutrients, they can be eliminated by soaking and proper preparation.

Therefore, legumes are a great plant-based source of protein.

37. Green beans

Green beans, also called string beans, are unripe varieties of the common bean. They are very popular in Western countries.

38. Kidney beans

Kidney beans are loaded with fiber and various vitamins and minerals. Make sure to cook them properly, as they're toxic when raw.

39. Lentils

Lentils are another popular legume. They're high in fiber and among the best sources of plant-based protein.

40. Peanuts

Peanuts (which are legumes, not a ae nuts) are incredibly tasty and high in nutrients and antioxidants. Several studies suggest that peanuts can help you lose weight.

However, take it easy on the peanut butter, as it's very high in calories and easy to overeat.

41–43: Dairy

For those who can tolerate them, dairy products are a healthy source of various important nutrients.

Full-fat dairy seems to be the best, and studies show that people who eat the most full-fat dairy have a lower risk of obesity and type 2 diabetes.

If the dairy comes from grass-fed cows, it may be even more nutritious — as it's higher in some bioactive fatty acids like conjugated linoleic acid (CLA) and vitamin K2.

41. Cheese

Cheese is incredibly nutritious, as a single slice may offer about the same amount of nutrients as an entire cup (240 ml) of milk. For many, it's also one of the most delicious foods you can eat.

42. Whole milk

Whole milk is very high in vitamins, minerals, quality animal protein, and healthy fats. What's more, it's one of the best dietary sources of calcium.

43. Yogurt

Yogurt is made from milk that's fermented by adding live bacteria to it. It has many of the same health effects as milk, but yogurt with live cultures has the added benefit of friendly probiotic bacteria.

44–46: Fats and oils

Many fats and oils are now marketed as health foods, including several sources of saturated fat that were previously demonized.

44. Butter from grass-fed cows

Butter from grass-fed cows is high in many important nutrients, including vitamin K2.

45. Coconut oil

Coconut oil contains relatively high amounts of MCTs, may aid Alzheimer's disease, and has been shown to help you lose belly fat.

46. Extra virgin olive oil

Extra virgin olive oil is one of the healthiest vegetable oils you can find. It contains heart-healthy monounsaturated fats and is very high in antioxidants with powerful health benefits.

47–48: Tubers

Tubers are the storage organs of some plants. They tend to contain a number of beneficial nutrients.

47. Potatoes

Potatoes are loaded with potassium and contain a little bit of almost every nutrient you need, including vitamin C.

They'll also keep you full for long periods. One study analyzed 38 foods and found that boiled potatoes were by far the most filling.

48. Sweet potatoes

Sweet potatoes are among the most delicious starchy foods you can eat. They're loaded with antioxidants and all sorts of healthy nutrients.

49. Apple cider vinegar

Apple cider vinegar is incredibly popular in the natural health community. Studies show that it can help low.er blood sugar levels and cause modest weight loss

It's great to use as a salad dressing or to add flavor to meals.

50. Dark chocolate

Dark chocolate is loaded with magnesium and serves as one of the planet's most powerful sources of antioxidants.

The bottom line

Whether you want to overhaul your diet or simply change up your meals, it's easy to add a number of these foods to your routine.

Many of the foods above not only make a great snack but are also packed with vitamins and antioxidants. Some of them may even aid weight loss.

If you don't normally challenge your palate, don't be afraid of trying something new.

www.ingramcontent.com/pod-product-compliance
Lightning Source LLC
Chambersburg PA
CBHW072330270726
48658CB00016B/2267